Instructor's Guide

for

Reading, Understanding, and Applying Nursing Research: A Text and Workbook

James A. Fain, PhD, RN, FAAN
University of Massachusetts Medical Center
Associate Professor and Director, Collaborative PhD Program in Nursing
Graduate School of Nursing
Worcester, Massachusetts

F. A. Davis Company
1915 Arch Street
Philadelphia, PA 19103

Printed in the United States of America

Last digit indicates print number: 10 9 8 7 6 5 4 3 2 1

Managing Publisher, Nursing: Lisa A. Biello
Acquisitions Editor: Joanne P. DaCunha, RN, MSN
Production Editor: Stephen D. Johnson
Cover Designer: Louis J. Forgione

As new scientific information becomes available through basic and clinical research, recommended treatments and drug therapies undergo changes. The author and publisher have done everything possible to make this book accurate, up to date, and in accord with accepted standards at the time of publication. The authors, editors, and publisher are not responsible for errors or omissions or for consequences from application of the book, and make no warranty, expressed or implied, in regard to the contents of the book. Any practice described in this book should be applied by the reader in accordance with professional standards of care used in regard to the unique circumstances that may apply in each situation. The reader is advised always to check product information (package inserts) for changes and new information regarding dose and contraindications before administering any drug. Caution is especially urged when using new or infrequently ordered drugs.

PREFACE

Most faculty would readily agree that a course in research methods belongs in a baccalaureate as well as a master's curriculum—as long as someone else teaches it! The reluctance of faculty to teach this subject is grounded in a variety of misconceptions and stereotypes:

- First, faculty believe they are not qualified enough to teach such a course. This attitude is based on the misconception that research is an activity done by a chosen few. For many faculty, their involvement in research has been limited to completing a master's thesis or doctoral dissertation.

- Second, many faculty have an understanding of research that is too narrow, too restricted. Because of their own educational backgrounds, they often understand research only in terms of rigid formulas, complicated budgets, and statistical expertise.

- These misconceptions in turn lead to a third reason for the reluctance of many faculty to teach research methods. One of the many common, but inaccurate, stereotypes is that faculty are uninterested in research. It is true that some faculty may view research as being less important compared with other required courses. However, the problem lies in what they perceive as a lack of relevancy of the research to clinical skills development. There is no reason why faculty and students alike should view research as being a "second-class" endeavor. Information related to research needs to be helpful and applicable to practice.

Reading, Understanding, and Applying Nursing Research: A Text and Workbook is intended to counteract or overcome all these roadblocks to the effective teaching of research to undergraduate as well as graduate students. The text provides information and strategies to help students understand, experience, and value research. Because the discipline of nursing continues to grow so rapidly with regard to both the knowledge it contains and the methodologies it employs, carefully defined goals is a first step in deciding how to approach the subject matter.

Goals and Objectives

Educators have discovered that curriculums take on greater clarity, direction, and purpose if they are described in terms of their intended goals and objectives. Goals are broad statements of what they hope to accomplish. Goals have an idealistic quality, inviting faculty to reflect on the course in terms of how it relates to student needs.

Objectives are statements that define how to get to the intended goals. Thus, objectives are more specific in terms of purpose than goals. By dealing with the nitty-gritty, objectives name the specific tasks that must be accomplished if the goals are to be achieved. In short, whereas goals speak to the course in its entirety, objectives clearly state what is to be accomplished and move students toward the desired goals.

The goals for *Reading, Understanding, and Applying Nursing Research: A Text and Workbook* are twofold:

- Provide students with the basic information needed to understand the research process, from idea conception through data analysis and interpretation.
- Enable students to use this knowledge to read and understand nursing research reports.

The objectives for the text, *Reading, Understanding, and Applying Nursing Research: A Text and Workbook,* are specified at the beginning of each chapter.

Organization of Textbook and Workbook

Reading, Understanding and Applying Nursing Research: A Text and Workbook is organized into fifteen chapters. The text emphasizes how to read research reports, how to evaluate them critically, and how to apply the findings to practice. The text is organized into three parts. In Part I, Nature of Research and the Research Process, the importance of nursing research is presented, and suggested research activities for nurses are presented in several documents. In Part II, Planning a Research Study, specific aspects of the research process are discussed from both a quantitative and qualitative approach. In Part III, Utilization of Nursing Research, suggested strategies for evaluating and critiquing research reports are introduced, along with guidelines for utilization of research findings.

The workbook was developed to accompany the text, *Reading, Understanding, and Applying Nursing Research: A Text and Workbook.* Therefore, each chapter in the workbook corresponds to a chapter in the text. There are three main sections associated with most chapters in the workbook: Review Questions, Multiple Choice Questions, and Critical Thinking Questions. Information in the workbook is designed to assist students in comprehending the content of each text chapter and in developing the ability to critique research reports.

Instructor's Guide

Like the workbook, each chapter in the *Instructor's Guide* corresponds to a chapter in the textbook and contains the following information:

Learning Objectives. Each chapter contains several objectives identifying specific behaviors the student is expected to exhibit as a result of the learning experience. Learning objectives are realistic, measurable, and attainable.

Answers to Review Questions. The workbook presents a set of review questions relevant to the information in each chapter. Answers to those questions are provided in the *Instructor's Guide.*

Answers to Multiple Choice Questions. The workbook presents a set of multiple choice questions relevant to the information in each chapter. Answers to those questions are provided in the *Instructor's Guide.*

Answers to Critical Thinking Questions. Most chapters of the workbook include a set of critical thinking questions. In some cases, excerpts from actual research reports are also presented to give students an opportunity to critique various sections. Answers to those critical thinking questions are provided in the *Instructor's Guide.*

Optional Resources. In some chapters, additional information is provided in preparing for a particular class.

Additional Exercises. Additional suggestions are also provided for activities to increase faculty-student interactions.

CONTENTS

PART I NATURE OF RESEARCH AND THE RESEARCH PROCESS

CHAPTER 1
Introduction to Nursing Research

LEARNING OBJECTIVES:

At the end of this chapter, you will be able to:

1. Describe the importance of nursing research for nurses.
2. Explain how the scientific method is applied in nursing research.
3. Describe the nurse's role as a consumer of research.
4. Identify strategies for executing research responsibilities.

ANSWERS TO REVIEW QUESTION:

1. Nursing research is essential to the development and refinement of knowledge used to improve clinical practice. As a practice discipline, nursing has developed its own unique body of knowledge that focuses on knowing, experiencing, and understanding individuals and their health experience.

2. For some students, a course in research is generally considered boring and approached with anxiety and apprehension. The term "research" conjures up an image of spending long hours in a library or laboratory. Many students are uneasy about the idea of research because of what they perceive as a lack of relevancy to clinical skills development. The focus of research should be on making research findings applicable and valuable to one's professional career. Research findings need to viewed as a vehicle for helping to determine the best way to improve clinical practice.

3. The problem-solving process is not synonymous with the research process. The problem-solving process involves identifying a problem and available options based on current knowledge. The research process involves discovering, validating, or generating new knowledge.

4. Ways of knowing within the discipline of **nursing come** from several different approaches. Chapter 1 provides the reader with an assortment of methods used to acquire knowledge (i.e., intuition, logical reasoning, tradition, practical experience, common sense, trial and error, and authority). Esthetic knowledge is another type of knowledge; it involves identification of patterns and includes analysis of phenomena that are perceived by the senses (i.e., what the nurse hears, sees, feels, smells). This is somewhat related to intuitive knowing. Because nursing is a practice discipline, both basic and applied knowledge are important to the discipline. Various types of knowledge are needed to understand the nursing care needs of individuals.

5. Scientific inquiry is different from other types of inquiry in that data are collected, analyzed, and reported.

6. Throughout the process of identifying and refining a research question, three general criteria should be considered to determine whether a questions is worth pursuing: the research question should be important, it should be answerable, and it should be feasible.

7. Students in a baccalaureate program need to be consumers of research with an ability to read, interpret, and evaluate research reports. In addition, they are responsible for sharing the results of research with colleagues. At the master's level, students are required to facilitate the conduct of research by collaborating in the development of an idea for a research project, assisting in data collection and analysis, and evaluating research findings for possible use in the practice setting.

8. Participating in a journal club; attending research presentations; serving as a member on an institutional review board.

9. *Cardiovascular Nursing*; *Heart & Lung*; *Journal of Pediatric Nursing*; *Maternal Child Nursing*; *Public Health Nursing*; *The Diabetes Educator*; *Home Care Nurse*; *Critical Care Nurse; Journal of Psychosocial Nursing; Archives of Psychiatric Nursing.*

ANSWERS TO MULTIPLE CHOICE QUESTIONS:

1. Nursing research is the key to providing high-quality health care. Through the research process, nurses
    a. ask questions that come up in daily nursing practice that need answers
    b. provide data that document the effectiveness of nursing care
    c. build a body of knowledge unique to the discipline of nursing
    d. all of the above
    d. is the correct answer

2. The scientific method incorporates those procedures used by researchers in the pursuit of new knowledge. The first step in the scientific method is:
    a. developing a framework
    b. reviewing the literature
    c. formulating a research problem and purpose
    d. formulating research objectives, questions, and/or hypotheses
    c. is the correct answer

3. Nursing has historically acquired new knowledge from an assortment of methods. Which of the following methods has nursing used to generate new ideas and knowledge?
   a. tradition
   b. personal experience
   c. intuition
   d. all of the above
   d. is the correct answer

4. An approach used to acquire nursing knowledge that describes life experiences is classified as:
   a. qualitative research
   b. quantitative research
   c. experimental research
   d. quasiexperimental research
   a. is the correct answer

5. Triangulation refers to the process of:
   a. reaching agreement among three members of a research team on the identity of the concepts or themes
   b. collecting data through different research approaches
   c. abstracting themes into constructs
   d. examining problems to gain knowledge about improving care to patients
   a. is the correct answer

OPTIONAL RESOURCES:

If you have time to read more information in preparation for this class, you might want to choose from the following:

American Nurses' Association: A Social Policy Statement.
    American Nurses' Association, Kansas City, MO, 1996.
Carper, BA: Fundamental patterns of knowing in nursing.
    Advances in Nursing Science 1:13, 1978.
Donaldson, SK, and Crowley, DM: The discipline of nursing.
    Nurs Outlook 26:113, 1978.
Newman, MA, Sime, AM, and Corcoran-Perry, SA: The focus of
    the discipline of nursing. Advances in Nursing Science
    14:1, 1991.

ADDITIONAL EXERCISE:

1. Students' familiarity with nursing research may vary considerably. Some may be familiar with the importance of nursing research and may even have been involved in the development of an idea for a research project; others will have virtually no experience. Allow the students to discuss their experience with research-related activities. Review and record their answers.

CHAPTER 2
Overview of the Research Process

LEARNING OBJECTIVES:

At the end of the chapter, you will be able to:

1. Identify the basic components of the research process.
2. Distinguish between basic and applied research; experimental and nonexperimental research.
3. Describe the process of ensuring that study participants have been protected from violation of human rights.
4. Define informed consent and its key elements.
5. Explain the role of institutional review boards in safeguarding the rights of subjects participating in a study.
6. Explain how to evaluate the ethical implications of a research report.

ANSWERS TO REVIEW QUESTIONS:

1. Selecting and defining the problem; selecting a research design; collecting data; analyzing data; using research findings.

2. Basic research is referred to as "pure research." Its major purpose is to obtain empirical data that can be used to develop, refine, or test a theory without immediate concern for direct application to clinical practice. Applied research is conducted to gain knowledge that can be used in a practical setting. In experimental research, the researcher manipulates and controls one or more variables and observes the effects in another variable(s). Nonexperimental research does not allow a strong degree of control over variables.

3. Retrospective research examines data collected in the past, whereas prospective research examines data collected in the present.

4. Cross-sectional research collects data at one point in time and draws conclusions about developments within a population, whereas longitudinal research collects data on a cohort of subjects over time.

5. The Nuremberg Code and Declaration of Helsinki were two documents that helped in the development of guidelines to ensure the protection of human subjects while conducting research. The Nuremberg Code addresses the protection of human rights by requiring informed consent. The Declaration of Helsinki outlines when participation in a research study would be harmful or of little value to subjects. On the basis of these two documents, the American Nurses' Association (ANA) developed two documents that provide specific directions for nurses engaged in research.

6. Right to freedom from injury; right to privacy and dignity; right to anonymity and confidentiality.

7. Anonymity refers to keeping individuals nameless, whereas confidentiality refers to protecting individuals and/or data by not divulging information gathered without permission.

8. Providing subjects with an estimate of the potential risks in relation to the potential benefits of a research study is referred to as the risk-benefit ratio.

9. Informed consent is providing individuals with sufficient information about participating in a
research study and with assurance that participation is voluntary and can be withdrawn at anytime without negative consequences.

10. The Committee for Protection of Human Subjects in Research. This committee, also known as the Human Subjects Committee (HSC), serves as the institutional Review Board (IRB) for our institution. The committee's functions and responsibilities are to ensure that all human subject research conducted at the institution is done according to ethical principles and that all research complies with the regulations described in Part 46 of Title 45 of the Code of Federal Regulations. The IRB membership consists of individuals representing diverse backgrounds and varying levels of scientific expertise. Membership is voluntarily. Meetings are held on the first and third Tuesday of each month, with additional meetings scheduled as necessary.

ANSWERS TO MULTIPLE CHOICE QUESTIONS:

1. The research process may best be characterized as:
    a. a way of assigning people to groups
    b. a set of steps to be carried out one by one in the prescribed order
    c. a set of rules that must always be followed
    d. a decision-making process in which attempts are made to guard against making false interpretations
    d. is the correct answer

2. In some situations, a researcher obtains informed consent without asking the subjects to sign their name on a written consent form. This may be done to protect the subjects'
    a. human dignity
    b. anonymity
    c. right to self-determination
    d. confidentiality
    b is the correct answer

3. Which of the following potential research participants have diminished autonomy and are incompetent to give informed consent?
   a. cognitively impaired older adults
   b. mentally ill patients
   c. children
   d. all of the above
   d. is the correct answer

4. A researcher wants to determine if nurses' levels of empathy for patients change after graduation from nursing school. She measures the following groups on empathy toward patients and compares their scores: new graduates, nurses who have worked for 2 years, and nurses who have worked for 4 years. This study is:
   a. prospective
   b. retrospective
   c. cross-sectional
   d. longitudinal
   c. is the correct answer

5. A researcher is interested in why some elderly patients are discharged when considered "not medically stable." The researcher reviews charts of patients who have been discharged in to explore factors that occurred during the hospitalization and relate these to status at discharge. This study is:
   a. prospective
   b. retrospective
   c. cross-sectional
   d. longitudinal
   b. is the correct answer

OPTIONAL RESOURCES:

If you have time to read more information in preparation for this class, you might want to choose from the following:

> Cassidy, VR, and Oddi, LF: Legal and ethical aspects of informed consent: A nursing research perspective. J Prof Nurs 2:343, 1986.
>
> Gleit, C, and Graham B: Secondary data analysis: A valuable resource. Nurs Res 38:380, 1989.
>
> Herron, DG: Secondary data analysis: Research method for the clinical nurse specialist. Clinical Nurse Specialist 3:66, 1989.
>
> Murphy, SA: Multiple triangulation: Applications in a program of nursing research. Nurs Res 38:294, 1989.
>
> Myers, ST, and Haase, JE: Guidelines for integration of quantitative and qualitative approaches. Nurs Res 38:299, 1989.
>
> Thompson, PJ: Protection of rights of children as subjects for research. J Pedi Nurs 2:393, 1987.

ADDITIONAL EXERCISE:

1. The basic ethical question for all researchers to consider is, "Will any physical or psychological harm come to anyone as a result of my research?" Ask the students to identify and discuss different sorts of ethical questions that might arise in their particular areas of interest? Have students briefly comment on how they would deal with these issues.

PART II PLANNING A RESEARCH STUDY

CHAPTER 3
Selecting and Defining the Problem

LEARNING OBJECTIVES:

At the end of this chapter, you will be able to:

1. Distinguish between a problem statement and purpose of the study.
2. List several characteristics of a good problem statement.
3. Identify a problem statement in a journal article.
4. Cite different sources of ideas for selecting a research problem.
5. Discuss the purposes of a literature review.
6. Identify the characteristics of a relevant literature review.
7. Differentiate between primary and secondary sources.
8. Compare advantages and disadvantages of print and computer database sources for searching the literature.

ANSWERS TO REVIEW QUESTIONS:

1. The problem statement consists of several paragraphs identifying a clinically researchable problem and citing significant literature sources to justify the study. The purpose statement usually follows the problem statement and is a single statement that identifies why the problem is being studied. The purpose statement likewise specifics the overall goal and intent of the research while clarifying the knowledge to be gained.

2. Characteristics of a problem statement include a researchable problem (able to collect and analyze data); operational definitions for variables or concepts within the study, and feasibility of conducting research on the problem.

3. A majority of research problems are derived from clinical practice.

4. Replication of research studies are an excellent way for researchers to discover results that conflict with previous research or disconfirm some aspect of an established theory. Some researchers believe that replication is less scholarly or less important than original research.

5. The literature review serves several purposes: discovers what has already been studied and/or what needs to be done; identifies gaps or inconsistencies within the literature; describes the strengths and weaknesses of previous research designs; and generates further research questions and/or hypotheses.

6. Three nursing research journals that contain empirical-based literature include *Nursing Research, Research in Nursing and Health, and Image: Journal of Nursing Scholarship.*

7. The discussion of previous research (literature review) within a research report can be as short as two or three sentences. Complete reviews of literature are usually not found in research articles because of page limitations.

8. Books are seldom referred to in a literature review because they tend to discuss a theoretical framework for the study. This is not say that the review of literature should be confined to published research reports. Subjective papers may be used as a source of important information that adds to an understanding of clinical content.

9. Primary sources of information are written by the person(s) who developed or generated the ideas published, whereas secondary sources are pieces of information summarizing or quoting content from the original or primary source.

10. Several important print indexes useful in nursing include the *International Nursing Index (INI)*, *Cumulative Index to Nursing and Allied Health Literature (CINAHL)*, *and Index Medicus (IM)*. Computer-based indexes include *Medline, Psychological Abstracts,* and *Educational Resource Information Center (ERIC)* database.

ANSWERS TO MULTIPLE CHOICE QUESTIONS:

1. The purpose of an operational definition is to:
    a. assign numerical values to variables
    b. specify how a variable will be defined and measured
    c. state the expected relationships among the variables under study
    d. designate the overall plan by which the research will be conducted
    b. is the correct answer

2. A review of literature serves several functions. They include:
    a. expanding or further defining your problem statement
    b. helping to establish a theoretical base
    c. identifying relationships among variables
    d. all of the above
    d. is the correct answer

3. A nurse decides to conduct a historical study about the care of chronically ill children in American frontier families between 1800 and 1820. Which of the following would be a primary source on this topic?
   a. Jones, *History of American West,* published in 1930
   b. a previous historical study, *The Nature of Childhood among Nebraska Settlers in the 1800s,* which was recently completed by a prominent nurse researcher
   c. a set of three letters, written by a pioneer woman in Minnesota from 1811 to 1812, concerning the experiences of her family, which included one child with asthma
   d. all of the above
   c. is the correct answer

4. As a nurse researcher you are studying the evolution of nursing and read the English translation of a book written by a Russian nurse. This source is:
   a. primary
   b. original
   c. secondary
   d. tertiary
   c. is the correct answer

5. Reproducing or repeating a study to determine whether similar findings will be obtained is referred to as:
   a. secondary research
   b. replication
   c. secondary analysis
   d. meta-analysis
   b. is the correct answer

ANSWERS TO CRITICAL THINKING QUESTIONS:

1. Identify pertinent background information leading to the proposed study.

    Paternal anxiety during a healthy pregnancy is common. With high-risk pregnancies paternal stress is increased. Activity restriction on mothers who are experiencing a high-risk pregnancy has recently been investigated. However, little information is available on how fathers respond to having their mates placed on bedrest during pregnancy. Some research findings have indicated that men frequently derive their primary source of support from their partners.

2. Provide information on the significance or importance of the proposed problem in relation to nursing.

    A high-risk pregnancy heightens both maternal and paternal stress. An estimated 700,000 women are placed on bedrest at home or in the hospital every year in efforts to reduce the prevalence of preterm births. Thus, health-care providers have focused their attention on the needs of the woman experiencing a high-risk pregnancy while giving little attention to fathers and their responses to this situation.

3. Based on the information provided within the problem statement and review of literature, evaluate the existing knowledge on the proposed problem.

    Results from research studies indicate that men experience high levels of worry, an overload of responsibility, and receive little if any attention from health-care providers. In addition, men exhibit depression and anxiety, with little perceived support.

4. Identify the gaps this study intends to fill.

    Further research is needed that addresses fathers' responses and the type of support they needed when their mates are placed on bedrest during most of their pregnancy.

5. What was the purpose or purposes of this study?

The purpose of this study was to describe the problems and stress of men whose pregnant partners are placed on bedrest and the assistance they received.

OPTIONAL RESOURCES:

If you have time to read more information in preparation for this class, you might want to choose from the following:

Beyea, SC, and Nicoll, LH: Writing an integrative review. AORN J 67:877, 1998.

Byrne, MM, Kangas SK, and Warren, N: Advice for beginning nurse researchers. Image: J Nurs Sch 28:165, 1996.

Gaberson, KB: What's the answer? What's the question? AORN J 66:148, 1997.

Ganong, LH: Integrative reviews of nursing research. Res Nurs Health 10:1, 1987.

ADDITIONAL EXERCISES:

1. To further explore the importance of conducting a comprehensive review of literature, divide the class into groups of four or five. Have each group identify a research question of interest. Each student is to find one reference on the question and make appropriate notes. Then have each group summarize the information and report back to the class. Several questions to be addressed during the discussion include: Has an in-depth review of literature been conducted on this topic? Have all sides of the problem been presented? How recent are the publications? Have primary sources been used?

2. Students may have a difficult time identifying the relevance of research to everyday problems faced by staff nurses in practice. Provide an opportunity for students to collaborate with staff in their clinical courses to identify nursing problems that need to be investigated. Discuss these problems in class. Several questions to be addressed during the discussion include: Are the problems "researchable"? Do theses problems focus on an area of concern to nursing?

CHAPTER 4
Formulating Hypotheses and Research Questions

LEARNING OBJECTIVES:

At the end of this chapter, you will be able to:

1. Define a hypothesis.
2. Identify characteristics of a hypothesis.
3. Write different types of hypotheses.
4. Compare and contrast inductive versus deductive hypotheses, directional versus nondirectional hypotheses, simple versus complex hypotheses, and statistical (null) versus research hypotheses.
5. Describe the appropriate use of research questions.
6. Define independent, dependent, and extraneous variables.

ANSWERS TO REVIEW QUESTIONS:

1. Hypotheses are statements that explain or predict relationships or differences among two or more variables in terms of expected results or outcomes of a study.

2. Hypotheses serve several purposes: guide scientific inquiry for the advancement of knowledge; provide direction for the research design and data collection, analysis, and interpretation; identify appropriate statistical analyses to be performed.

3. Hypotheses should state clearly and concisely the expected relationships (or differences) among two or more variables. In addition, each hypothesis should address a single relationship (or difference) that is testable. Likewise, variables identified in hypotheses must be operationally defined.

4. Directional hypotheses are usually derived from conceptual models or previous literature indicating a direction to the relationship between variables under study.

5. Studies in which prior knowledge on a particular area of study is limited contain research questions, and the purpose of these study seeks to identify or describe the phenomena.

6. Hypotheses are never proved true or false. Hypotheses are either supported (accepted) or not supported (rejected).

7. Hypotheses are evaluated by statistical analyses. The type of statistical analysis depends the level of measurement associated with each variable(s) being studied.

8. No significant difference will exist between blacks and whites with type II diabetes on self-reported dietary adherence.

9. Complex directional hypothesis.

10. An independent variable is observed, introduced, or manipulated by the researcher to determine the effect it has on another variable. Independent variables are sometimes referred to as "predictor variables," "treatment variables," or "experimental variable." A dependent variable is observed for change or reaction after the treatment application. The dependent variable is determined by the researcher as the result of conducting a study. Dependent variables are sometimes referred to as "criterion" or "outcome" variables. An extraneous variable is a one that confounds the relationship between the independent and dependent variable. Extraneous variables are sometimes referred to as "confounding variables."

ANSWERS TO MULTIPLE CHOICE QUESTIONS:

1. An example of a directional hypothesis is:
   a. Persons with dementia who receive an orienting intervention will show less confusion and fewer problem behaviors than those who do not receive the orienting intervention.
   b. There will be no difference in maternal and infant outcomes between women birthed in a hospital and those birthed at home while cared for by a midwife.
   c. There will be a difference in weight among persons who have attended a nutrition program compared with those who have not attended the program.
   d. Those patients receiving total parenteral nutrition who have a hydrocolloid dressing versus a standard gauze dressing will show differences in the incidence of catheter-related infection and local inflammation at the insertion site.

   a. is the correct answer.

2. Patients with type II diabetes who receive instruction on an individual basis will be more compliant than those who receive instruction in a group setting." Identify the dependent variable in this hypothesis.
   a. type II diabetes
   b. individual versus group setting
   c. compliance
   d. type of instruction

   c. is the correct answer

Questions 3 and 4 refer to the example below:

You are concerned that subjects presenting to the emergency room with nonemergency problems are not following through on recommended referrals. You believe that you can influence this by incorporating systematic patient teaching into the visit, so you design a teaching intervention. Persons who present to the emergency room with urinary tract infection are randomly assigned to receive or not receive the teaching intervention; those not receiving the intervention are given a short written handout containing instructions to follow-through on referral.

3. The independent variable is:
   a. urinary tract infections
   b. emergency room
   c. follow-through on referral
   d. teaching intervention
   d. is the correct answer

4. From the list below, which would you suggest for use as a dependent variable in this study?
   a. education of the nurse
   b. education of the subject
   c. making an appointment with the referral agency
   d. presence or absence of urinary tract infection
   c. is the correct answer

5. Control techniques are introduced to reduce the contaminating effects of:
   a. independent variable
   b. extraneous variables
   c. dependent variables
   d. null hypotheses
   b. is the correct answer

ANSWERS TO CRITICAL THINKING QUESTIONS:

1. Identify the independent variable and dependent variable in hypothesis I.

    Independent variable = Implementation of strategies to promote independence in dressing (SPID); those residents receiving the intervention (experimental group) versus those not receiving the intervention (control group)

    Dependent Variable = ability to dress independently

2. How would you classify hypotheses I and II?

    Hypothesis I: Simple directional hypothesis
    Hypothesis I: Null hypothesis

3. Identify the population being studied in hypotheses I and II.

    Nursing home residents who are cognitively impaired (CI)

4. Rewrite hypothesis II to state a relationship between the variables.

    Nursing assistants who complete the SPID will be able to complete dressing activities of the cognitively impaired (CI) nursing home resident in less time compared with those nursing assistants who do not participate in the SPID.

OPTIONAL RESOURCES:

If you have time to read more information in preparation for this class, you might want to choose from the following:

Beyea, SC, and Nicoll, LH: What is a variable? AORN J 66:500, 1997.

Machoyeanos, MK: The hypothesis: Its use and meaning. Matern Child Nurs J 22:215, 1997.

ADDITIONAL EXERCISE:

1. Have students identify several examples of hypotheses using research journals or specialty journals that publish research reports. Ask students to identify the independent and dependent variables. Discuss whether any extraneous (confounding) variables are apparent? Which variables listed in the hypotheses need to be operationally defined?

CHAPTER 5
Selecting the Sample and Setting

LEARNING OBJECTIVES:

At the end of this chapter, you will be able to:

1. Define a sample and a population.
2. List the characteristics, uses, and limitations of each kind of probability and nonprobability sampling.
3. Distinguish between random selection and random assignment.
4. Discuss the importance of a representative sample.
5. Define external validity.

ANSWERS TO REVIEW QUESTIONS:

1. The population for a study is often referred to as the target population, whereas an accessible population is some portion of the target population that is readily available to the research study from which the sample is selected.

2. A sample is representative of the population when individuals selected to be in a study are characteristic of the larger group (target population).

3. Sampling procedures ensure that the sample chosen is representative of the larger group (target population). A representative sample places researchers in a stronger position to draw conclusions form the sample findings that are generalizable to the target population. However, there are no guarantees, regardless of which sampling procedures are used.

4. A sampling frame is a list of all subjects, objects, events, or units in the population.

5. A table of random numbers is used to conduct a random selection of subjects, objects, events, or units.

6. A researcher makes inferences about a population on the basis of knowledge drawn from the sample.

7. Random selection is the equal, independent chance of individuals being selected for a study and refers to a method used to choose study participants. Random assignment is the random allocation of subjects to either an experimental or a control group.

8. Several types of probability sampling include simple random sampling, stratified random sampling (disproportional and proportional), cluster sampling (multistage), and systematic sampling.

9. A majority of published research reports use nonprobability sampling because of the difficulties in obtaining random access to populations.

10. External validity is the extent to which study results can be generalized from the study sample to other subjects, populations, and settings.

ANSWERS TO MULTIPLE CHOICE QUESTIONS:

1. The population from which the researcher selects the research sample is commonly referred to as:
   a. target population
   b. universal population
   c. accessible population
   d. available population
   c.   *is the correct answer*

2. Which of the following sampling methods provides a sample that is most representative of the target population?
    a. simple random sampling
    b. convenience sampling with random assignment to groups
    c. quota sampling
    d. purposive sampling
    a. is the correct answer

3. Another name for probability sampling is:
    a. accidental
    b. random
    c. quota
    d. purposive
    b. is the correct answer

4. A nurse practitioner (NP) in a primary care clinic decides to study the health promotion practices of her patients. The NP makes a list of all adult patients seen in the clinic for the past 6 months. There are 475 patients on the list. By assigning a number to each name and using a table of random numbers, the NP selects 100 patients to be invited to participate in the study. What type of sample has been selected?
    a. simple random sample
    b. stratified random sample
    c. convenience sample
    d. purposive sample
    a.   is the correct answer

5. You are shopping in the mall and are approached by a researcher for a local food chain. The researcher asks you to participate in a study by answering a few questions. As a study participant, you were selected by which method of sampling?
   a. random
   b. convenience
   c. systematic
   d. network
   b. is the correct answer

ANSWERS TO CRITICAL THINKING QUESTIONS:

1. What type of sampling technique was used in this study? Identify its strengths and weaknesses.

    Nonprobability sampling was the technique used to recruit women into the study. Nonprobability sampling usually requires less time with an accessible population. However, with nonprobability sampling, the ability to generalize the findings becomes an issue, because the sample chosen may not represent the larger target population.

2. Describe some of the sample characteristics.

    Seventy-nine women consented to participate in the study. The sample ranged in ages from 25 to 85 years (mean [M] = 54.9, standard deviation [SD] = 28.6); 37% of the sample was older than 60 years. A majority of the subjects were white (83.5%), married (70%), and well educated (M = 14.7 years, SD = 2.4 years). Forty-four percent were employed outside the home, with 51% having an annual income over $50,000.

3. What was the general procedure for recruiting subjects into the study?

    Women were recruited from a large urban tertiary care center. Women were considered eligible to participate if they were English speaking, received a first diagnosis of cancer within the past 3 to 7 months, and were 21 years of age or older. No other specific data collection procedures were reported.

4. State the significance of the following statement: "Demographic and clinical characteristics of the refusers were statistically similar to those of the study sample?"

    There was no difference between those women who agreed to participate in the study and those women who did not agree to participate (refusers) in terms of demographic and clinical characteristics.

OPTIONAL RESOURCES:

If you have time to read more information in preparation for this class, you might want to choose from the following:

Beyea, SC, and Nicoll, LH: Selecting samples for research studies requires knowledge of the population of interest. AORN J 66:722, 1997.

Diekmann, JM, and Smith, JM: Strategies for access and recruitment of subjects for nursing research. West J Nurs Res 11:418, 1989.

Timmerman, GM: The art of advertising for research studies. Nurs Res 45:339, 1996.

ADDITIONAL EXERCISES:

1. To illustrate sample selection, ask students to identify an area of interest and the population to be studied. Then, instruct students to outline a method for selecting a random sample from that population. Have students describe the type of sampling method they chose and why.

2. Help students understand that no sampling technique guarantees a representative sample. Using real or fictitious data, select a random sample using three methods: (a) drawing names from a hat, (b) flipping a coin, and (c) using a table of random numbers. Compare the characteristics of the sample chosen by the three methods as to how representative each sample is of the population. For example, if 25% of the population was female, which sampling method was closest to 25%? How would you explain that answer?

CHAPTER 6
Principles of Measurement

LEARNING OBJECTIVES:

At the end of this chapter, you will be able to:

1. Compare and contrast the four types of scales of measurement.
2. Discuss the issue of reliability, and distinguish among the various types.
3. Discuss the issue of validity, and distinguish among the various types.
4. Discuss the relationship between reliability and validity.

ANSWERS TO REVIEW QUESTIONS:

1. The nominal level of measurement is the lowest level of measurement that consists of assigning numbers as labels for categories. These numbers have no numerical interpretation. An ordinal level of measurement specifies the order of items being measured without specifying how far apart they are. Ordinal scales classify categories incrementally and rank-order each category. Interval levels of measurement possess all characteristics of a nominal and an ordinal scale, in addition to having equal interval sizes based on an actual unit of measurement. Ratio levels of measurement are the highest level of measurement and are characterized by equal distances between scores with an absolute zero point.

2. Blood type (i.e., A, B, AB, O) is a nominal level of measurement.

3. Observations on a nominal scale cannot be converted to an interval/ratio scale. However, observations on an interval/ratio scale can be converted to a nominal scale. Higher levels of measurement can be converted to lower levels; however, the reverse is not true.

4. Reliability = consistency.

5. The coefficient of stability, also referred to as test-retest reliability, deals with the consistency of repeated measurements. It is the degree to which scores are consistent over time.

6. One of the more popular statistical procedures used to assess internal consistency is Cronbach's alpha coefficient. This procedure is used to assess internal consistency when instruction items are scored categorically (i.e, 1 to 4). Another statistical procedure used to assess internal consistency is called Kuder-Richardson #20, or simply, KR-20. This procedure is used when the items of an instrument are scored dichotomously (i.e., 1 for yes; 0 for no).

7. In some studies, researchers collect data by having raters evaluate a particular situation. Cohen's kappa statistic is used to quantify the degree of consistency among raters.

8. Validity is the accuracy with which an instrument or a test measures what it is suppose to measure.

9. Factor analysis (an advanced statistical procedure) is a popular method used to assess construct validity.

10. The process of determining validity is by no means an easy task. An instrument may have excellent reliability, but not measure what it claims to measure. However, an instrument's data must be reliable if they are to be valid. Thus, high reliability is a necessary, though insufficient, condition for high validity.

ANSWERS TO MULTIPLE CHOICE QUESTIONS:

1. Which of the following measurements is at the ratio level?
   a. self-rating on the following scale: nonsmoker, light smoker, heavy smoker
   b. religious affiliation
   c. minutes of second-stage labor
   d. age defined as: individuals younger than 25 years old and those older 26 years old
   c. is the correct answer

2. As a teacher you rank a group of students from most competent to least competent. Which type of scale has been described?
   a. nominal
   b. ordinal
   c. interval
   d. ratio
   b. is the correct answer

3. Variables that consist of just two categories are referred to as:
   a. dichotomous
   b. continuous
   c. linear
   d. alpha
   a. is the correct answer

4. Cronbach's alpha is used to determine which of the following instrument attributes?
   a. test-retest reliability
   b. internal consistency reliability
   c. interrater reliability
   d. stability
   b is the correct answer

5. Instrument reliability and validity are related to each other in which of the following ways?
   a. an instrument that is not valid cannot be reliable
   b. an instrument that is not reliable cannot be valid
   c. reliability and validity are completely independent characteristics
   d. reliability and validity are completely interdependent; that is, if an instrument is reliable it is also valid

   a. is the correct answer

ANSWERS TO CRITICAL THINKING QUESTIONS:

1. The following is a list of variables. How each variable is defined is located within the brackets. Identify the appropriate level of measurement for each variable.
   a. sleep problems: [absence or presence of sleep problems] *nominal*
   b. birth weight of a neonate: [in grams] *interval/ratio*
   c. type of solution for intravenous replacement: [crystalloid versus colloid] *nominal*
   d. amount of vacation: [actual number of days] *interval/ratio*
   e. height: [in terms of percentile] *ordinal*

   Questions 2 and 3 deal with excerpt from the literature:

2. What type of reliability is discussed in the excerpt. Are the reliability coefficients at an acceptable level. Explain your answer.
   Internal consistency was assessed by using Cronbach's alpha coefficients. The AIDS/HIV Knowledge Scale had a high internal consistency of .85 (pretest) and .93 (post-test). In addition, the AIDS Risk-Taking Behavior Scale demonstrated fair alpha coefficients of .77 (pretest) and .74 (post-test). Likewise, fair test-retest reliabilities were reported for both scales (.79 at 2-month interval for the AIDS/HIV Knowledge Scale; .73 at 2-month interval for the AIDS Risk-Taking Behavior Scale). It is typical for affective measures to have stability reliabilities in the high .80s or low .90s.

2. How would a researcher go about assessing content validity on the measures described in the excerpt?

Typically, instruments (i.e., AIDS/HIV Knowledge Scale and AIDS Risk-Taking Behaviors Scale) are developed from concepts in the literature that reflect a range of dimensions associated with the variable being measured. Content validity is assessed by a panel of experts. Individuals with expertise in the area of acquired immunodeficiency syndrome/human immunodeficiency (AIDS/HIV) would be chosen to review the appropriateness of items within the scales. These experts would review the scale and make suggested changes, additions, and deletions.

OPTIONAL RESOURCES:

If you have time to read more information as a preparation for this class, you might want to choose from the following:

Gaberson, KB: Measurement reliability and validity. AORN J 66:1092, 1997.

Machoyeanos, MK: Methods for assessing the accuracy of measuring instruments. Matern Child Nurs J 21(pt I):311, 1996.

Machoyeanos, MK: Methods for assessing the accuracy of measuring instruments. Matern Child Nurs J 22(pt II):53, 1997.

Munro, BH: Statistical Methods for Health Care Research, ed 2. JB Lippincott, Philadelphia, 1997, p 310.

ADDITIONAL EXERCISES:

1. Provide the students with a list of variables (i.e., anxiety, pain, socioeconomic status, hope, family support). Ask students to operationally define the variables at the ordinal and interval/ratio levels of measurement.

2. It is pointed out in this chapter that scores from an instrument may be reliable but not valid, yet not the reverse. Review once again with students why this is so.

3. Review with students the type of evidence each of the following examples represents with respect to content, criterion-related, and construct validity.

    a. Ninety-five percent of students who score high on a research methods examination receive A's as end-of-semester grades in research.

    b. A professor of nursing looks over a test that measures student knowledge of research methods and states that, in his or her opinion, the test measures such knowledge.

    c. A professor discovers that students who score high on a particular test on quantitative versus qualitative approaches to research also receive high marks in the research course. The professor also finds out that these same students are rated high among clinical faculty who ask students to write a paper focusing on the application of research findings to practice.

CHAPTER 7
Data Collection Methods

LEARNING OBJECTIVES:

At the end of this chapter, you will be able to:

1. Identify common instruments and methods used to collect data in quantitative and qualitative research.
2. Distinguish between closed-ended and open-ended questionnaires.
3. List the advantages and disadvantages of using questionnaires.
4. Compare and contrast the different types of scaling techniques.

ANSWERS TO REVIEW QUESTIONS:

1. Data collection methods used by researchers to collect quantitative data include surveys and questionnaires, scales, and biophysical measures. Data collection methods used by researchers to collect qualitative data include interviews with possible use of audio/video recordings and participant observation.

2. Closed-ended questionnaires ask subjects to select an answer from among several choices. This type of questionnaire is often used in large surveys when questionnaires are mailed. Open-ended questionnaires ask subjects to provide specific answers. This type of questionnaire allows participants to write a response as opposed to answer a question with fixed choices. It is less frequently found in studies in which quantitative methods for data analysis are planned.

3. Some guidelines to follow when designing a questionnaire include using simple language, having each question represent just one idea, delimiting any reference to time, and phrasing questions in a neutral way.

4. Questionnaires are often mailed to subjects participating in a study. A concern with use of questionnaires is the response rate. When only a small percentage of subjects return questionnaires, it may be unreasonable to assume that those who did respond were typical of the group as a whole. Response rates of 60% to 80 % are considered excellent.

5. The response-set bias is the amount of measurement error introduced by the tendency of some individuals to respond to items in characteristic ways (i.e., always agreeing/disagreeing) independent of the item's content.

6. Likert-type scales and semantic differential scales are similar in that subjects are asked to read a statement of pair of adjectives and select an appropriate ranked response (i.e., the response is assigned a value from 1 to 7).

7. A psychosocial instrument is a paper-and-pencil test that measures a particular psychosocial concept or variable.

8. By reverse scoring, original values associated with specific items on an instrument are reversed (i.e., items originally scored as 7 should be reversed to be 1; 6=2, 5=3, 4=4, 3=5, 2=6, and 1=7).

9. A visual analogue scale (VAS) is a 100-mm-line-long scale, with anchors at each end to indicate extremes of the phenomenon being assessed. Subjects are asked to mark a point on the line indicating the amount of the phenomenon experienced at a particular point in time.

10. Several biophysical measures include vital signs (i.e., temperature, pulse, respirations, blood pressure), maximum inspiratory pressure, cardiac output, glycosylated hemoglobin, urine catecholamine levels, and coagulation tests).

ANSWERS TO MULTIPLE CHOICE QUESTIONS:

1. Which of the following data collection procedures provide "richer" data?
   a. searches through medical records or files
   b. observational techniques
   c. self-administered questionnaires
   d. structured interviews
   a. *is the correct answer*

2. The use of questionnaires in research has many advantages. They include all of the following *except*:
   a. facilitates collecting data from large samples
   b. associated with good response rates
   c. easily coded and tabulated
   d. expense of printing is considerably less than interviewing
   a. *is the correct answer*

3. Several different response formats are available when using Likert scales. The most popular response choices address issues of:
   a. agreement
   b. frequency
   c. importance
   d. all of the above
   d. *is the correct answer*

4. On a 7-point Likert scale, the response "undecided" would probably be scored as:
   a. 0
   b. 1
   c. 4
   d. 7
   b. *is the correct answer*

5. If subjects are not very verbal or articulate, which type of data
   collection method would be most appropriate?
   a. open-ended questionnaire
   b. closed-ended questionnaire
   c. unstructured interview
   d. use of a diary to keep field notes
   b. is the correct answer

ANSWERS TO CRITICAL THINKING QUESTIONS:

1. Were the steps in collecting data described clearly and concisely?
Explain your answer.
    *Data collection procedures were explained clearly and
    concisely. The research report indicated that nurses working in the
    oncology and radiation department reviewed records to determine
    whether women receiving treatment for breast cancer met eligibility
    criteria. A convenience sample of women were invited to participate
    in the study. At either a regularly scheduled appointment in the clinic
    or over the telephone, the nurse researcher described the study and
    told the women what would be expected of them if they decided to
    participate.*

2. Was the instrument (i.e., Psychosocial Adjustment to Illness Scale
   [PAIS]) used to collect data appropriate based on the purpose of the
   study? Explain your answer. Were issues of reliability and validity
   discussed?
    *From what is presented in this short excerpt, the PAIS
    appeared to be an appropriate measure based on the purpose of the
    study (examining the relationship between self-blame and illness
    adjustment among women with breast cancer). Issues of reliability
    were assessed by Cronbach's alpha coefficients (i.e., r = .63 and .67).
    The article speaks of these reliabilities as being high Many
    researchers would consider high reliabilities as those in the high .80s
    or low .90s. The issue of construct validity was assessed by the
    statistical procedure factor analysis.*

3. Was the PAIS described as to how it was scored? range of possible scores? What does a high or low score mean?

A more detailed discussion of the PAIS is warranted after reading this short excerpt. The authors state that the PAIS is a 46-item semistructured interview. Are all 46 items closed ended? The potential range for the PAIS is 0 to 184, with higher PAIS scores indicating poorer adjustment. Mention of subscales are reported? How many items make up each subscale? How are these subscales scored? Do you report both a total PAIS score and individual subscale scores?

OPTIONAL RESOURCES:

If you have time to read more information in preparation for this class, you might want to choose from the following:

Bernal, H, and Wooley, S, and Schensul, JJ: The challenge of using Likert-type scales with low-literate ethnic populations. Nurs Res 46:179, 1997.

Gable, RK, and Wolf, MB: Instrument Development in the Affective Domain, ed 2. Kluwer Associates, Boston, 1993.

Waltz, CF, Strickland, OL, and Lenz, ER: Measurement in Nursing Research, ed 3. FA Davis, Philadelphia, 1991.

ADDITIONAL EXERCISE:

1. Review with students the various types of data collection methods discussed in the chapter. Of all the methods presented, which one(s) do ou think would be the hardest to use? the easiest? Which one(s) do you think would provide the most dependable information? Why?

CHAPTER 8
Analyzing the Data

LEARNING OBJECTIVES:

At the end of this chapter, you will be able to:

1. Differentiate between descriptive and inferential statistics.
2. Compare and contrast the three measures of central tendency.
3. Compare and contrast the three measures of dispersion.
4. Distinguish between parametric and nonparametric procedures.
5. Evaluate a researcher's choice of descriptive and inferential statistics in published research.

ANSWERS TO REVIEW QUESTIONS:

1. The three most commonly used measures of central tendency are mean (M), median, and mode. The mean is very sensitive to outliers, or extreme values.

2. The three most commonly used measures of dispersion are range, variance, and standard deviation (SD). The range is the simplest measure of dispersion to calculate.

3. Two distributions can have the same mean but a different standard deviation. Kurtosis refers to a measure of "peakedness" or "flatness" as it relates to the distribution of a given sample. In a flat distribution, the standard deviation is larger. In a narrow (peakedness) distribution, the standard deviation is smaller.

4. Probability is an essential concept for understanding inferential statistics and refers to the researcher's ability to predict.

5. A level of confidence is a probability level that is established by a researcher. The .05 level of confidence is accepted by most researchers in all sciences; that is, researchers are willing to accept statistical significance occurring by chance 5 times out of 100.

6. The Pearson Product-Moment Correlation *(r)* is a common correlational coefficient that examines the relationship between two variables. Correlational coefficients greater than $r = .70$ are considered acceptable.

7. A correlational coefficient of $r = -.78$ indicates a stronger correlation when compared with $r = +.53$.

8. Researchers use independent *t*-test when scores in one group have no logical relationship with scores in the other group. A second type of *t*-test is termed dependent *t*-test (also referred to as matched *t*-test, correlated *t*-test) and is used when scores in the first group can be paired with scores in the second group. The classic example is when a subject contributes two scores, one pretest score and one post-test score. Both scores are paired and have a logical relationship with one another.

9. *t*-Tests and analysis of variance (ANOVA) are similar in that the analysis is based on mean scores.

10. Two types of chi-square (x^2) include one-sample x^2 (sometimes referred to as "goodness-of-fit" test) and independent samples x^2 test.

ANSWERS TO MULTIPLE CHOICE QUESTIONS:

1. As a researcher you collect data on the marital status of your clients. The appropriate measure of central tendency to use for this variable is:
   a. mean
   b. median
   c. mode
   d. standard deviation
   c. is the correct answer

2. The appropriate measure of dispersion for the above example is:
   a. range
   b. variance
   c. standard deviation
   d. none of the above
   d. is the correct answer

3. On what basis does the *t*-test compare groups?
   a. frequency distributions
   b. mean score
   c. alpha level
   d. confidence intervals
   b. is the correct answer

4. Which of the following correlation coefficients would give you the most precise prediction?
   a. $r = .80$
   b. $r = -.60$
   c. $r = .45$
   d. $r = -.85$
   a.   is the correct answer

5. In an analysis of variance (ANOVA), for the F ratio to be significant, the between-group variances should be:
   a. about the same as the within-group variance
   b. about the same as the probability level
   c. larger than the within-group variance
   d. smaller than the within-group variance
   c. is the correct answer

ANSWERS TO CRITICAL THINKING QUESTIONS:

1. As a researcher you are interested in using the Jalowiec Coping Scale (JCS). The JCS consists of a list of 20 coping behaviors derived from a comprehensive review of literature. Ten items are classified as "problem oriented" and 10 items are classified a "affective oriented" behaviors. Degree of use of behaviors is rated on a 1- to 5-point Likert scale with descriptive endpoints of "never" and "almost always." Subjects are asked to estimate how often they use various behaviors to cope with stress. You conduct a pilot study using the JCS on a group of graduate students. The following data represent the students' scores on the JCS:

   61, 58, 22, 96, 95, 21, 20, 35, 22, 92, 26, 42, 52, 26

   a. Calculate the following descriptive statistics with respect to the prior distribution of JCS scores: mean, median, mode, range, variance, standard deviation.

M = 47.71	*Range = 20 to 96*
Median = 38.5	*Variance = 828.53*
Mode = 22 and 26	*SD = 28.78*

b. Using the data calculated above, write three of four sentences describing the JCS scores using measures of central tendency and dispersion.

> *The mean of the distribution of JCS scores was 47.71 (SD = 28.78), with a range of 20 to 96. The median of the distribution was 38.50. There is a difference between the mean and median indicating a skewed distribution. Terms such as skewness and kurtosis are used to describe characteristics of the shape of the distributions. The terms describe how or where the frequencies of scores are concentrated. Likewise, the distribution is bimodal, indicating that two scores occur more frequently than other scores.*

1. Subjects were recruited from a list of patients who had undergone a cardiac catheterization after being admitted to the hospital with a diagnosis related to cardiac disease. Two groups of patients were identified: those who attended a postdischarge coronary artery disease (CAD) education class held at the institution (intervention group) during an 8-month period immediately before data collection and those who had not attended the class (comparison group). Health-promoting behavior was measured with the Health-Promoting Lifestyle Profile (HPLP). The HPLP is a 48-item questionnaire composed of six subscales that measure the frequency of self-reported health-promoting behaviors in several domains. Total scores and subscale scores are derived by summing the respective responses. Higher scores indicate more frequent performance of health-promoting behavior. Means and standard deviations (SDs) for the HPLP total score and subscales by each group are presented in the following table.

Mean and Standard Deviation of Health-Promoting Behavior Scales by Group

	Intervention		Comparison		t
	M	SD	M	SD	
Total HPLP	140.7	20.57	129.64	22.24	2.55*
Subscales					
Self-actualization	41.76	6.83	39.31	7.93	1.69
Health responsibility	27.75	5.22	24.25	6.06	3.11*
Exercise	12.02	4.41	11.30	4.41	0.87
Nutrition	19.42	3.47	17.29	3.68	3.10*
Interpersonal support	21.57	3.94	20.16	4.18	1.78
Stress management	19.69	3.91	18.38	3.85	1.60

Source: Plach, S., Wierenga, M.E., and Heidrich, S.M. Effect of postdischarge
      education class on coronary artery disease knowledge and self-reported health-
      promoting behaviors. Heart & Lung 25:367, 1996.
*$p < 0.01$

1. What type of *t*-test was computed in the above example: independent
   or dependent *t*-test? Explain your answer.
        Independent t-*test were calculated. Independent* t-*tests are
   *used when one group (intervention) has no logical relationship to the
   other group (comparison).*

2. On the basis of the *t*-test analyses shown in the previous table, describe
   the findings in two or three sentences.
        *On the basis of the findings reported in the table, those
   individuals in the intervention scored significantly higher on the total
   HPLP (140.7 versus 129.64) as well as on the subscales health
   responsibility (27.75 versus 24.25) and nutrition (19.42 versus 17.29)
   when compared with individuals in the comparison group.*

3. Is the following hypothesis supported or not supported based on the
   findings presented in the table: "Patients who attend the CAD
   education class will report more interpersonal support compared with
   those patients who do not attend the CAD education class." Explain
   your answer.

This hypothesis is not supported based on results presented in the table. There was no significant differences on the interpersonal support score between those in the intervention group versus those in the comparison group.

Optional Resources:

If you have time to read more information in preparation for this class, you might want to choose from the following:

Brogan, DR: Choosing an appropriate statistical test of significance for a nursing research hypothesis of question. West J Nurs Res 3:337, 1981.

Holm, K, and Christman, NJ: Post hoc tests following analysis of variance. Res Nurs Health 8:207, 1985.

LeFort, SM: The statistical versus clinical significance debate. Image: J Nurs Sch 25:57, 1992.

Oberst, MT: Clinical versus statistical significance. Cancer Nurs 5:475, 1982.

Siegel, S, and Castellan, NJ: Nonparametric Statistics for the Behavioral Sciences, ed 2. McGraw Hill, New York, 1988.

ADDITIONAL EXERCISE:

1. Clinical information is a rich source of research data. Interest in using clinical information for research purposes has increased among clinicians and researchers alike. Provide students with some type of clinical database, large or small. Have students identify the level of measurement associated with each variable (i.e., nominal, ordinal, interval/ratio) within the database. Describe the database by calculating appropriate measures of central tendency and dispersion.

CHAPTER 9
Selecting a Research Design:
Quantitative versus Qualitative

LEARNING OBJECTIVES:

At the end of this chapter, you will be able to:

1. Understand the links between philosophy and research questions, with regard to selection of design.
2. Define and explain the purpose of research design.
3. Describe characteristics of a good research design.
4. Compare and contrast significant quantitative and qualitative aspects of research designs.
5. Understand a selected group of designs from both a quantitative and qualitative perspective.
6. Appreciate the process that underlies research design selection.

ANSWERS TO REVIEW QUESTIONS:

1. Quantitative research is directed at the discovery of relationships and cause and effect. In addition, quantitative research refers to measurement and analysis of causal relationships among variables. Qualitative research is directed at discovery of meaning rather than cause and effect. Qualitative research involves the use of language, concepts, and words, rather than numbers, to represent evidence from research.

2. Characteristics of a good research design are evident when the following attributes are well grounded: evidence of the fit between philosophy, theory, and data collected; the purpose, or focus, of the study is reflected in the type of design chosen; and the level of concept development and knowledge advancement matches the type of research design chosen.

3. Control is very important in quantitative research, especially when constructing experimental designs. Control refers to those elements or techniques built into a research design to reduce or eliminate interpretations of the cause of results. Use of randomization into an experimental or control (comparison) group is an example of control. The concept of control in a qualitative study has little significance. The research design is more flexible, to attain a more comprehensive understanding of phenomena in a naturalistic setting.

4. A true experimental design is an experiment in which the researcher tries to assess whether an intervention or treatment makes a difference in a measured outcome. The following elements are present in all true experimental designs: control, random assignment, and manipulation of the independent variable. In quasiexperimental designs, random assignment and/or a control group are not necessary. Often nurse researchers will use a quasiexperimental design because of the nature of the study or clinical setting. It may be difficult or impossible to use a control group or randomly assign patients to groups based on the nature of the study.

5. The most basic type of quasiexperimental design is the nonequivalent control group design. This type of design in also referred to as a comparison group, with no randomization of subjects.

6. Subjects in an experimental group receive a particular intervention, whereas subjects in a control group do not receive the intervention. Outcomes are measured in both groups and compared.

7. In an experiment, the independent variable is manipulated. The independent variable is sometimes referred to as the intervention or treatment.

8. Internal validity refers to whether or not the independent variable actually made a difference. True experimental designs usually have a high degree of internal validity because of the use of control groups and randomization. Several threats to internal validity include history, maturation, testing, instrumentation, statistical regression, and mortality.

9. Descriptive designs gather information about conditions, attitudes, or characteristics of individuals or groups of individuals. An advantage of a descriptive design is the ability to describe the meaning of existing phenomena. No attempt is made to control or manipulate the variables under study.

10. Secondary analysis uses previously collected data to test new hypotheses, explore new relationships, or create new insights. Meta-analysis is a statistical technique that uses the findings from several studies to create a data set that may be analyzed as a single piece of data.

ANSWERS TO MULTIPLE CHOICE QUESTIONS:

1. A concern researchers have about a qualitative approach to research is:
   a. the need for larger sample sizes
   b. the lack of fit with questions relevant to nursing
   c. the lack of rigor in its methodologies
   d. the time-consuming nature of its methodologies
   a.   *is the correct answer*

2. In choosing a quasiexperimental design over a true experimental design, the researcher realizes that the study would involve less:
   a. bias
   b. control
   c. rigor
   d. significance
   b. is the correct answer

3. What threat to internal validity is being controlled for when a researcher completes an experiment in a relatively short time to minimize developmental changes?
   a. history
   b. maturation
   c. testing
   d. instrumentation
   b. is the correct answer

4. What threat to internal validity is being controlled when a researcher uses reliable and valid assessment tools or scales for rating or scoring to avoid biases?
   a. history
   b. maturation
   c. testing
   d. instrumentation
   d. is the correct answer

5. In meta-analysis, the sample consists of:
   a. incidents occurring to a single subject
   b. research instruments
   c. previous studies
   d. human subject
   c. is the correct answer

ANSWERS TO CRITICAL THINKING QUESTIONS:

1. Describe the type of research design appropriate for this study based on the research questions posed. Explain your answer.

   Each of the three research questions gather information about a particular condition (i.e., pattern of occurrence of symptoms, number of patients requiring analgesic medication, and amount of time after surgery that patients can resume normal eating and living patterns). Thus, a descriptive research design is appropriate. In each example, there is no manipulation of variables.

2. What are the advantages and disadvantages of the design listed in question 1.

   An advantage of the descriptive design is one of reporting information that has not been noted in previous literature. A disadvantage of this type of design is the inability to manipulate the independent variable or impose any types of control in the design.

OPTIONAL RESOURCES:

If you have tune to read more information in preparation for this class, you might want to choose from the following:

Beyea, SC, and Nicoll, LH: Qualitative and quantitative approaches to nursing research. AORN J 66:323, 1977.

Grey, M: Experimental and quasiexperimental designs. In LoBiondo-Wood, G, and Haber, J (Eds): Nursing Research: Methods, Critical Appraisal, and Utilization, ed 4. Mosby-Year Book, St. Louis, 1998, pp 175–193.

Marcus, PR, and Liehr, PR: Qualitative approaches to research.. In LoBiondo-Wood, G, and Haber, J (Eds): Nursing Research: Methods, Critical Appraisal, and Utilization, ed 4. Mosby-Year Book, St. Louis, 1998, pp 215–245.

ADDITIONAL EXERCISES:

1. Have the students identify the difficulties in meeting the criteria of a true experimental design.

2. Specific threats to internal validity depend on the type of design and generalizations the researcher hopes to make. Have the students critique an assigned article that illustrates an experimental or a quasiexperimental design. Discuss whether more than one threat to internal validity is found in the study. If there is only one, can a study have more than one threat to internal validity? Does finding a threat to internal validity invalidate the results of the study? How does the researcher handle this type of finding?

CHAPTER 10
Phenomenological Research

LEARNING OBJECTIVES:

At the end of this chapter, you will be able to:

1. Define phenomenology.
2. Discuss phenomenology as a philosophy and a research method.
3. Discuss phenomenological research methods.
4. Differentiate phenomenological research methods from other qualitative research.
5. Describe the relevance of phenomenology to nursing research and practice.
6. Review and critique phenomenological research in nursing.

ANSWERS TO REVIEW QUESTIONS:

1. Phenomenology is a qualitative research approach applicable to the study of phenomena that influences nursing practice. In phenomenological terms, this is referred to as the "lived experience." The purpose of phenomenology is to describe the intrinsic traits, or essences, of the lived experience.

2. Bracketing requires the researcher to identify any previous knowledge, ideas, or beliefs about the phenomena under investigation. Intuiting refers to the researcher being immersed in the descriptions of the lived experience, to acquire a comprehensive and accurate interpretation.

3. The researcher needs to become totally immersed in the phenomenon under investigation. The researcher becomes the tool for data collection and listens attentively to each individual throughout the interview process. The researcher then studies the data as they are transcribed and reviews them over and over again.

4. It is common to use a small, purposive sample of individuals who have lived and are willing to describe the experience under study. Saturation refers to the participants' descriptions becoming repetitive with no new or different ideas or interpretations emerging.

5. The primary data-collecting techniques used in phenomenological research include interviewing participants and written descriptions of the lived experience.

6. Ethical considerations and informed consent issues are the same whether a researcher is conducting quantitative or qualitative research.

7. Scientific rigor is documented in qualitative research by suggesting confirmability associated with the data. Confirmability has three elements: (a) auditability: requires the reader of qualitative research to be able to follow the decision path of the researcher in arriving at certain findings; (b) credibility: requires that findings are faithful descriptions or interpretations of the lived experience; and (c) fittingness: requires that the study findings fit the data; that is, findings are grounded in the lived experience under study and reflect the typical and atypical elements of that experience.

8. Data analysis exists in phenomenological research when the researcher engages into a dialogue with the data and uses inductive reasoning and synthesis. A system to file, code, and retrieve data is a necessary first step. Early transcription and analysis of tape-recorded interviews are essential.

9. Hermeneutics is a research method or strategy that focuses on language and written text to capture the essence of the lived experience.

10. The greatest strength of phenomenological research is the ability to uncover and explore everyday experiences.

ANSWERS TO MULTIPLE CHOICE QUESTIONS:

1. The basic aim of a phenomenological study is to:
   a. study individuals, artifacts, or documents in their natural setting
   b. study social data for the purpose of explaining some phenomenon
   c. study the nature or meaning of everyday experiences
   d. study the cause and effect relationships among variables
   a. is the correct answer

2. In phenomenological research, researchers must acknowledge any previous information, ideas, or beliefs about a particular phenomenon before proceeding with the study. This is referred to as:
   a. bracketing
   b. intuiting
   c. confirmability
   d. intentionality
   a. is the correct answer

3. Sampling in phenomenological research is:
   a. random
   b. purposive
   c. stratified
   d. quota
   b. is the correct answer

4. Data is collected in a phenomenological study through a variety of techniques, which include:
a. observation
b. descriptions written by subjects
c. unstructured interviews
d. all of the above
d. is the correct answer

5. The process of analyzing data in phenomenological research involves:

    a. computation
    b. thinking
    c. enumeration
    d. analytic memos
    b. is the correct answer

ANSWERS TO CRITICAL THINKING QUESTIONS:

1. Describe how the researcher became immersed in the data. What techniques did the researcher use to help participants describe meaning in their lives?

    The researcher became immersed in the data by conducting in-depth, face-to-face interviews lasting 1 to 2 hours. Follow-up interviews were performed to provide support and clarify meanings of statements. In addition, the researcher kept detailed field notes and a methodological journal to keep track of observations, decisions, and feelings.

2. The issue of trustworthiness in qualitative research is a concern for researchers engaging in these methods. How did the researcher address trustworthiness and authenticity of data?

    Issues of trustworthiness and authenticity of data were addressed by examining the elements of audibility, credibility, and fittingness. The notion of intuiting and reflecting on each transcribed tape provides evidence for audibility. There was, however, no mention of bracketing. The use of several interviews to clarify meaning provides evidence for credibility.

3. What is meant by the phrase, "collaborative discussion or hermeneutic conversations."

    Several members of the research team meet to discuss and reflect on the written text of each interview. Collectively, a greater understanding of the common themes, based on language used to capture the lived experience emerged.

OPTIONAL RESOURCES:

If you have time to read more information in preparation for this class you might want to choose from the following:

Beck, CT: Qualitative research: The evaluation of its credibility, fittingness, and auditability. West J Nurs Res 15:263. 1993.

Beck, CT: How students perceive faculty caring: A phenomenological study. Nurse Educator 6:18, 1991.

Cohen, MZ: A historical overview of the phenomenological movement. Image: J Nurs Sch 19:31, 1987.

Drew, N: The interviewer's experience as data in phenomenological research. West J Nurs Res 11:431, 1989.

Ornery, A: Phenomenology: A methods for nursing research. Advances in Nursing Science 5:49, 1983.

Reeder, F: The phenomenological movement. Image: J Nurs Sch 19:150, 1987.

Zalon, ML: Pain in frail, elderly women after surgery. Image: J Nurs Sch 29:21, 1997.

ADDITIONAL EXERCISE:

1. Phenomenology as a research approach provides an opportunity for researchers to describe the lived experience. Nurses in practice can be a tremendous source of data that has yet to he explored. Ask students to identify a type phenomenon unique to nursing practice that is important to the ever-expanding body of nursing knowledge. Have students discuss how they would know when data saturation has occurred. Possibly they can use examples from their own clinical experiences.

Chapter 11
Ethnographic Research: Focusing on Culture

LEARNING OBJECTIVES:

1. Identify a historical perspective of an ethnography and its use in nursing.
2. Describe major characteristics of ethnographic research.
3. Outline three stages of an ethnographic research study.
4. Delineate major findings from an ethnography in relation to a specific culture or subculture.
5. Identify potential applications of ethnographic research to nursing practice.

ANSWERS TO REVIEW QUESTIONS:

1. An ethnography is a qualitative research approach, developed by anthropologists, involving the study of individuals, artifacts, or documents in the natural setting. The researcher is involved in the data collection process and seeks to understand fully how life unfolds for the individual or group under study.

2. Ethnographic research has its roots in anthropology.

3. Ethnographic data are collected in the field. Fieldwork is an approach that involves prolonged residence with members of the culture being studied.

4. The first nurse researcher to become interested in ethnography as a research method was Madeline Leininger. Her interest in culture began to emerge while working as a child psychiatric mental health nurse.

5. As a participant observer, the researcher enters into the everyday life and activities of the people of the culture being studied. By watching what goes on, talking with individuals, and participating in activities, the researcher comes to know the culture shared by a particular group. Researchers may supplement their observations with a wide variety of data collection tools (i.e., key informant interviews, collection of life histories, structured interviews, questionnaires, documents, photographs).

6. Researchers tend to reside in the field for about a year, although the exact time frame has varied from as little as 8 months to as long as 5 years.

7. The planning and implementing of an ethnographic research study takes place in three stages: pre-fieldwork, fieldwork, and post-fieldwork.

8. The primary data collection technique used in ethnographic research is fieldwork aimed at describing and understanding a specific culture.

9. Researchers may supplement their observations with a wide variety of data collection tools, which include key informant interviews, collection of life histories, structured interviews, questionnaires, documents, and photographs.

10. Ethnography offers a research approach for the individual who is interested in learning about culture, willing and able to report data in narrative format, comfortable with ambiguity, and able to build trusting relationships. The study of culture offers exciting opportunities for discovery relevant to nursing practice.

ANSWERS TO MULTIPLE CHOICE QUESTIONS:

1. Ethnographic research can be characterized as a means of:
   a. studying the social psychological problems present within human interactions
   b. studying the lives, ways, or patterns of groups of individuals
   c. studying the events, ideas, institutions, or people to assess historical meaning
   d. all of the above

   b. is the correct answer

2. The planning and implementing of an ethnographic study takes place in three stages. During phase 1 of fieldwork, the researcher focuses on:
   a. developing trust and acceptance
   b. forming long-term relationships
   c. gathering information as is relates to the problem
   d. obtaining large amounts of information

   a. is the correct answer

3. What group of social scientists has the greatest interest and commitment to discovery of cultural knowledge?
   a. anthropologists
   b. psychologists
   c. sociologists
   d. philosophers

   a. is the correct answer

4. Observations recorded about the people, places, and things that are part of the ethnographer's study of a culture are referred to as:
   a. ethnographic styles
   b. genealogies
   c. field notes
   d. participant observers

   c. is the correct answer

5. The phrase "researcher as instrument" is a fundamental characteristic of ethnography. This refers to:
   a. the researcher's focusing on a combination of quantitative and qualitative methods of data collection
   b. the researcher's becoming immersed in direct observation and learning from members of cultural groups
   c. the process of data analysis whereby statements are grouped and given codes for ease of identification
   d. the degree of dedication a researcher commits to analyzing data collected during a qualitative study
   b. is the correct answer

ANSWERS TO CRITICAL THINKING QUESTIONS:

1. How did the researcher gain access to the culture being studied?
   The researcher gained access to participants in this study by participating in several activities with both mother or father and child (i.e., attending summer camp; going to restaurants; watching television). In addition, the researcher kept an ethnographic log and conducted several in-depth interviews with each family over a 1-year period.

2. Describe the various types of techniques used to collect data.
   Participant observation; in-depth interviews; ethnographic log.

OPTIONAL RESOURCES:

If you have time to read more information as preparation for this class, you might want to choose from the following:

Atkinson, P, and Hammersley, M: Ethnography and participant observation. In Denzin, NK, and Lincoln, YS (Eds): Handbook of Qualitative Research. Sage Publications, Thousand Oaks, CA, 1994, pp 248–261.

Geertz, C: The Interpretation of Culture. Basic Books, New York, 1973.

Miller, MP: Factors promoting wellness in aged person: An ethnographic study. Advances in Nurs Science 13:38, 1991.

Spradley, JP: Participant Observation. Holt, Rinehart & Winston, 1980.

ADDITIONAL EXERCISES:

1. Ask the students to identify a particular phenomenon that focuses on an ethnographic approach to research. Have the students discuss potential research questions. Remember, ethnographic nursing studies address questions that relate to how cultural knowledge, norms, and values influence one's health experience.

2. An ethnographer selects a cultural group that is living the phenomenon under investigation. The researcher gathers information from key informants. Have the students discuss what is meant by the term "key informants." Like phenomenologists, do ethnographers make their own beliefs explicit and bracket their personal biases as they seek to understand the culture of others?

CHAPTER 12
Grounded Theory Research

LEARNING OBJECTIVES:

At the end of this chapter, you will be able to:

1. Discuss symbolic interactionism as the theoretical framework of grounded theory.
2. Describe the steps in the research process for grounded theory.
3. Compare and contrast theoretical sampling with statistical sampling.
4. Explain the constant comparative method of data analysis.
5. Describe the difference between substantive and theoretical coding.
6. List criteria that can help a researcher decide on a core category.
7. Identify at least six families of theoretical codes.
8. Discuss criteria for judging grounded theory.
9. Distinguish between a core category and a basic social process.

ANSWERS TO REVIEW QUESTIONS:

1. Grounded theory is a qualitative research method based on the symbolic interactionist perspective of human behavior. Grounded theory research combines inductive and deductive research methods. With the use of inductive processes, theory emerges from the data. Deduction is then used to test theory empirically.

2. Grounded theory research has its roots in sociology. The original work of symbolic interaction is traced back to two sociologists from the University of Chicago, George Herbert Mead, and his student, Herbert Blumer. Symbolic interaction focuses on the nature of social interaction among individuals.

3. Participant observation, informal interviewing, and formal interviewing are the three main sources of data collection. Unstructured observational data are gathered in the field through a process called "participant observation." Like everyday conversations, informal interviewing can take a few minutes to more than an hour. Formal interviewing is used when the researcher wishes more in-depth information.

4. Theoretical sampling is the process of data collection for generating theory, whereby the researcher collects, codes, and analyzes data and then decides what data to collect next in order to develop the grounded theory. Theoretical sampling is done to discover categories. Unlike statistical sampling, a predetermined sample size is not calculated. In theoretical sampling, sample size is determined by generated data and analyzed until categories are saturated.

5. The constant comparative method of data analysis is a form of qualitative data analysis that makes sense of data by categorizing units of meaning by constantly comparing incidents until categories and concepts emerge. Substantive coding is the first stage of constant comparative data analysis, in which the initial discovery of categories occurs. Substantive coding is made up of open and selective coding. Open coding occurs when data are broken down into incidents and examined for similarities and differences. Selective coding begins only after the researcher is sure the core variable has emerged. To code selectively for a core variable means to delineate only variables that relate to the core variable.

6. The goal of grounded theory research is to generate a theory around a core category. A core category represents a pattern of behavior that is relevant and/or problematic for persons involved in a study.

7. In a grounded theory study, the review of literature does not occur at the start of a study. The grounded theorist begins by collecting data in the field and generating a theory. When the theory appears to be sufficiently grounded and developed, the literature in the field is reviewed and related to the developing theory. By waiting to complete a literature review, the researcher avoids contaminating the data with preconceived concepts that may or may not be relevant.

8. Memos are write-ups of ideas as they emerge while the grounded theorist is coding for categories. Memos are written as they strike the grounded theorist while he or she is constantly comparing, coding, and analyzing the data. The length of a memo can vary from a sentence, paragraph, or several pages.

9. Four criteria are used to judge the rigor of grounded theory: fit, work, relevance, and modifiability. Fit refers to the categories identified by the emerging theory corresponding to the data collected. Work involves indicating that the grounded theory explains what happens, predicts what will occur, and interprets an area of substantive or formal inquiry. To achieve relevance, the area of study must be relevant and comprehensible to individuals in the setting. The generation of theory is always being modified. A grounded theory can never be more correct than its ability to work the data. As new data reveal themselves in research, the theory is modified.

10. Grounded theory research plays a significant role in the conduct of qualitative research in that it can increase midrange substantive theories and help to explain theoretical gaps between theory, research, and practice. The method explores the richness of human experience by sharing a specific social psychological problem.

ANSWERS TO MULTIPLE CHOICE QUESTIONS:

1. Grounded theory is an important research method in that:
   a. theory is discovered to explain a particular phenomenon
   b. an accurate interpretation describes a particular phenomenon under study
   c. the meanings of actions and events are described by researchers seeking to understand a particular phenomenon
   d. all of the above
   d. is the correct answer

2. In grounded theory research, the research question(s) is:
   a. refined by the researcher as the data emerge
   b. identified by the researcher after the problem statement
   c. identified by an existing theory
   d. formulated based on the focus of the study
   a. is the correct answer

3. Data gathered in grounded theory research using field techniques, observational methods, and documents are examined and analyzed through a system referred to as:
   a. selective coding
   b. constant comparative method
   c. memoing
   d. trustworthiness
   b. is the correct answer

4. The process of data analysis in grounded theory whereby statements are grouped for ease of identification is referred to as:
   a. categorizing
   b. memoing
   c. coding
   d. theoretical analysis
   a. is the correct answer

5. The process of selecting concepts that have proven relevance to the evolving theory is known as:
   a. categorizing
   b. memoing
   c. coding
   d. theoretical analysis
   c. is the correct answer

ANSWERS TO CRITICAL THINKING QUESTIONS:

The following questions refer to Excerpt 12.1:

1. What is the substantive area of study in this grounded theory research study?
   Theory of parental coping processes

2. Why does the phenomenon of interest require a qualitative approach?
   Recurrence of cancer among children has been studied from a biological perspective. Little has been written on the impact and coping processes among parents when faced with such a crisis. To date, only anecdotal reports have suggested that parental coping is particularly difficult on parents. A qualitative study is appropriate to explore how parents cope with cancer recurrence in their children.

The following questions refer to Excerpt 12.2:

1. What strategies did the researchers use to analyze the data?
   Tape-recorded semistructured interviews, observations, and review of medical records. In addition, the three principal investigators shared transcribed interviews at their respective sites.

2. How did the researcher address the fit, credibility, and relevance of the research?

Fit *was addressed by constantly reviewing major themes using open and selective coding. Likewise, a review of memos was established after each interview. In assessing credibility and relevance, typed transcripts were shared with parents to check for accuracy before analyzes were conducted.*

OPTIONAL RESOURCES:

If you have time to read more information in preparation for this class, you might want
to choose from the following:

Bright, MA: Making place: The first birth in an intergenerational family context. Qualitative
Health Research 2:75, 1992.
Hutchinson, S: Grounded theory: The method. In Munhall, PL, and
Oiler, CJ (Eds): Nursing Research: A Qualitative Perspective.
Appleton-Century-Crofts, Norwalk, CT, 1986, pp 111–130.
Stem, PN: Grounded theory methodology: Its uses and processes. Image:
J Nurs Sch 12:20, 1980.
Turner, MA, Tomlinson, PS, and Harbaugh, BL: Parental uncertainty in
critical care hospitalization of children. Matern Child Nurs J 19:45, 1990.

ADDITIONAL EXERCISES:

1. An important aspect of grounded theory research is the fact that theory is connected to or "grounded in" the data. Have the students discuss what is meant by the phrase grounded in?

3. Ask the students to debate why the grounded theory method is appropriate when researchers are interested in social processes from the perspective of human interactions. Have the students also discuss why grounded theory research does not include the use of hypotheses

PART III   UTILIZATION OF NURSING RESEARCH

CHAPTER 13
Interpreting and Reporting Research Findings

LEARNING OBJECTIVES:

At the end of this chapter, you will be able to:

1. List factors to consider when interpreting research findings.
2. Explain how to interpret results and discuss findings of a study.
3. Distinguish between statistical and clinical significance.
4. Describe a logical sequence for writing a research report.
5. Identify methods of disseminating research findings.

ANSWERS TO REVIEW QUESTIONS:

1. Statistical significance indicates that the findings from an analysis are unlikely to be the result of chance. However, interpretation of findings must make logical sense and be clinically relevant. Achieving statistical significance does not automatically guarantee that a study has clinical value.

2. An essential part of evaluating results of a study is generalizability, or the extent to which research findings can be extended beyond the given research situation to other settings and subjects. Thus, it is essential to provide a detailed description of the sample characteristics so that the results can be generalized to those individuals.

3. The major goal of preparing a research report is to summarize key aspects of a study and to share the results with other researchers and colleagues.

4. Key aspects of a research report include the title, abstract, introduction (purpose and review of literature), methods (sample setting, data collection), results, discussion, and implications for practice.

5. An abstract is a concise and succinct summary of a research report. A well-written abstract provides an overview of the key aspects of a research report.

6. A well-written methods section allows other researchers to replicate the study.

7. Common mistakes to avoid when preparing a research report are described, but this description needs to be included in each of the major section of the research report. The problem statement should provide an understanding of the problem under study and be quickly followed by the purpose statement. The methods section should provide information on the research design, setting, sample, and data collection procedures and instruments. The results section should answer the research question(s) or test hypotheses. The discussion section should focus on a nontechnical interpretation of the results, or what the results mean in relation to the purpose of the study.

8. Disseminating research findings can be done through publications, oral presentations, and poster presentations.

9. The purpose of a query letter is to determine if the editor has an interest in reviewing a manuscript for possible publication.

10. A refereed journal is a peer-reviewed journal for which experts in the field review manuscripts and make recommendations to editors.

ANSWERS TO MULTIPLE CHOICE QUESTIONS:

1. Generalizability refers to:
   a. the extent to which findings from an analysis are unlikely to be the result of chance
   b. the extent to which research findings are reported objectively
   c. the extent to which statistical significance is related to clinical significance
   d. the extent to which results of a study can be applied to other people, instruments, and settings
   c. is the correct answer

2. Name the place in the research report where you would expect to find the following statement: "The purpose of this study was to examine the relationship between caregiver burden and social support among spouses of individuals with multiple sclerosis."
   a. introduction
   b. methods
   c. results
   d. discussion
   a.   is the correct answer

3. Name the place in the research report where you would expect to find the following statement: "Caregiving burden was measured using the Caregiving Burden Scale (CBS). The CBS is a list of 14 tasks that may be required of caregivers. These tasks are divided into three areas: direct care tasks, instrumental care tasks, and interpersonal care tasks."
   a. introduction
   b. methods
   c. results
   d. discussion
   b.   is the correct answer

4. Name the place in the research report where you would expect to find the following statement: "Subjects were 49 caregivers (25 women and 24 men) who were caring for adult family members receiving outpatient chemotherapy at a midwestern cancer center."
   a. introduction
   b. methods
   c. results
   d. discussion
   c. is the correct answer

5. Disseminating nursing research findings can be accomplished through:
   a. publications
   b. oral presentations
   c. poster presentations
   d. all of the above
   d. is the correct answer

ANSWERS TO CRITICAL THINKING QUESTIONS:

1. How concise and succinct is the abstract?
   The abstract is very concise and succinct, identifying the study's purpose, sampling technique, and results of correlational analyzes and hierarchical regression.

2. Does the title of the article capture the essence of the study. Explain your answer?
   The title captures the essence of the study by focusing on the specific problem and population being studied.

OPTIONAL RESOURCES:

If you have time to read more information in preparation for this class, you might want to choose from the following:

> Beyea, SC, and Nicoll, LI-I: Writing and submitting an abstract. AORN J 67:273, 1998.
>
> Beyea, SC, and Nicoll, LH: Developing and presenting a poster presentation. AORN J 67:468, 1998.
>
> Fain, JA: Writing an abstract. The Diabetes Educator 24:353, 1998.
>
> Morin, KH: Poster presentation: Planning. Matern Child Nurs J 21:206, 1996.
>
> Morin, KH: Poster presentation: Getting your point across. Matern Child Nurs J 21:307, 1996.
>
> Tornquist, EM: From Proposal to Publication: An Informal Guide to Writing about Nursing Research. Addison-Wesley, Menlo Park, CA, 1986.

ADDITIONAL EXERCISES:

1. Dissemination of research findings is the responsibility of all researchers. It is also important for researchers to know with whom to share the results. Ask the students to identify several research articles and address whether the audience or readership of the particular journal is appropriate based on the type of content and/or methodologies featured. Discuss whether there are research journals that publish more qualitative versus quantitative research.

2. Presenting research in a poster format is a challenge. Anyone who has ever attended a poster session knows that the volume of posters limits interested parties from spending time with each one. The poster must capture the attention of the reader immediately. Have each student identify a research article and display its contents in a poster format. Discuss ways to present information in an appealing way.

CHAPTER 14
Critiquing Research Reports

LEARNING OBJECTIVES:

At the end of this chapter, you will be able to:

1. Distinguish between a research critique and research review.
2. Apply principles that make a critique constructive rather than destructive.
3. Incorporate a set of guidelines in the critique of research reports.

ANSWERS TO REVIEW QUESTION:

1. A research review focuses on the major aspects of a study, summarizing its major features. A research critique goes beyond describing a particular study and critically evaluates the piece of research.

ANSWERS TO MULTIPLE CHOICE QUESTIONS:

1. Critiquing published research reports is important because it helps to:
   a. provide an increased understanding of the research process
   a. determine whether findings associated with a study are suitable for use in practice
   b. learn from other researchers and build on previous research
   d. all of the above
   d. is the correct answer

2. Individuals who critique published research reports should attempt to:
   a. focus on the inadequacies inherent in the study
   b. be as objective as possible
   c. evaluate the scientific merit of a study based on the researcher's credentials
   d. restrict the amount of critical comments that would discourage the researcher

   b. is the correct answer

3. A reviewer asks the question, "Is the problem being studied conceived as a nursing problem." Where in the research report should this question be addressed?
   a. problem statement
   b. methodology
   c. results
   d. discussion

   a. is the correct answer

4. A reviewer asks the question, "Are the analysis and interpretations of data adequate for the problem being studied?" Where in the research report should this question be addressed?
   a. problem statement
   b. methodology
   c. results
   d. discussion

   c. is the correct answer

5. A reviewer asks the question, "How will the results of this study be incorporated into practice?" Where in the research report should this question be addressed?
   a. problem statement
   b. methodology
   c. results
   d. discussion

   d. is the correct answer

CHAPTER 15
Research Utilization

LEARNING OBJECTIVES:

At the end of this chapter, you will be able to:

1. Define research utilization.
2. Describe the purpose of research utilization.
3. Identify the various methods of nursing research utilization.
4. Contrast the differences between research and research utilization.
5. Describe the steps of the research utilization process.
6. Discuss barriers and facilitators to the research utilization process.
7. Discuss strategies to promote the utilization of research into practice.

ANSWERS TO REVIEW QUESTIONS:

1. Research utilization is the process by which knowledge generated from a research study becomes incorporated in clinical practice.

2. Disseminating research findings provides an opportunity to develop research-based policies, procedures, and clinical guidelines to improve patient outcomes.

3. Nursing research utilization models were developed to enable the use or dissemination of nursing research. Historically, there has been a gap between research and clinical practice. Some research findings have been adopted by clinicians; other findings have never been incorporated into practice.

4. Knowledge diffusion is the process by which new information becomes part of practice and subject to evaluation.

5. Improving patient outcomes is the ultimate goal of nursing research utilization models. However, the target population, structure, and process may be different based on the type of nursing research utilization model. The Conduct and Utilization of Research in Nursing (CURN) Project's target population is a group of individuals interested in the same practice issue. The structure is institution based with the outcome focusing on changes in patient outcomes. The Stetler model focuses on the individual practitioner making decisions about the applicability of research findings. The Stetler model assists practitioners with research utilization evaluation.

6. Phases associated with the research utilization process include (1) specifying the problem, (2) assembling the literature, (3) critiquing the research, (4) assessing applicability, (5) implementing the innovation, and (6) evaluating the innovation.

7. The phrase "gap between research and practice" refers to the fact that research findings are not incorporated into practice. Nursing research is of little value unless the knowledge generated is incorporated into practice.

8. Barriers to research utilization are classified as research related (i.e., absence of research in a particular area, lack of experience reading research reports); professional and administrative (i.e., lack of time, money, clinical resources); and clinician barriers (i.e., not valuing or understanding how research utilization differs from conducting research).

9. Factors that enhance research utilization include identifying clinically relevant problems in practice, establishing journals clubs, increasing funding opportunities, sponsoring conferences and presentations that promote research utilization, creating rewards and recognition for implementing innovations, and targeting specific individuals in administration to lead the change process.

10. With the increasing interest in cost and quality of health care, research-based care will continue to be mandated in today's health-care market.

ANSWERS TO MULTIPLE CHOICE QUESTIONS:

1. Research utilization is a process by which:
   a. information generated from research becomes incorporated into practice
   b. researchers critically evaluate the importance of the phenomenon being studied
   c. researchers recognize the effectiveness of collaborating on research-related issues
   d. researchers develop project-specific outcome measures that are measurable
   a. is the correct answer

2. The primary focus of the Stetler model for research utilization is to facilitate application of
   research findings at what level?
   a. systems based
   b. practitioner
   c. institution based
   d. professional organization
   b. is the correct answer

3. Regardless of which nursing research utilization model is chosen, the first step in the research utilization process is:
   a. critiquing the literature
   b. identifying the problem
   c. implementing a change
   d. evaluating the change
   b. is the correct answer

4. Which of the following strategies for utilization is most amenable for students and staff nurses?
   a. replicating previous research studies
   b. reading and understanding published research reports
   c. preparing an integrative review of literature or meta-analysis
   d. devoting a specific amount of time to working with an established researcher
   b. is the correct answer

5. Which of the following is a barrier to research utilization?
   a. absence of research that explains practice
   b. lack of time, money, and clinical resources
   c. attending conferences outside your institution where research is presented
   d. establishing linkages between academics and practice professionals
   b. is the correct answer

OPTIONAL RESOURCES:

If you have time to read more information in preparation for this class, you might want to choose from the following:

> Beyea, SC, and Nicoll LH: Barriers to and facilitators of research utilization in perioperative nursing practice. AORN J 65:830, 1997.
>
> Bostrom, J, and Wise, L: Closing the gap between research and practice. J Nurs Admin 24:22, 1994.
>
> Cronenwett, LR: Effective methods for disseminating research findings to nurses in
>
> practice. Nurs Clin North Am 30:429, 1995.
>
> Gift, A: Nursing research utilization. Clinical Nurse Specialist 8:306, 1994.
>
> Prevost, SS: Research-based practice in critical care. Clinical Issues in Critical Care Nursing 5:101, 1994.

ADDITIONAL EXERCISES:

1. The conduct of research is of little value unless the findings are used in practice to improve the quality of patient care. Ask the students to identify one or two research articles in which the information is appropriate for application to practice. Discuss the current state of practice on a particular nursing unit with respect to the problem identified? Discuss how students might influence the behavior of nurses to let go of ritual-based practices and benefit from research-based protocols or standards.